A Young Adult Male's Guide to

Pleasure

Mastering

Sex
Positions

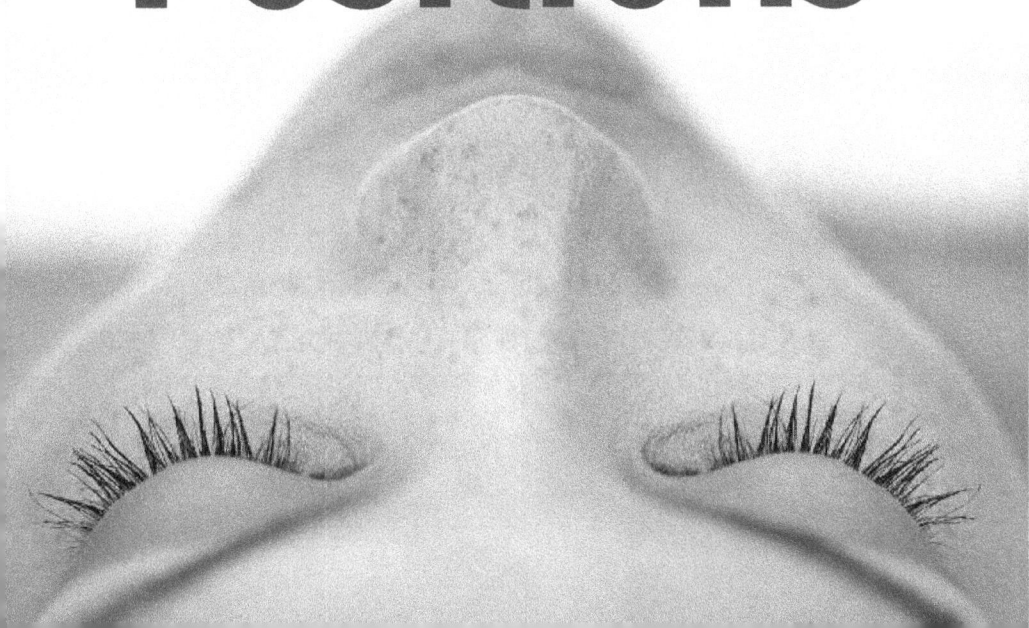

Table Of Contents

Chapter 1: Introduction
to Sexual Pleasure   4

Understanding Male
Sexual Anatomy   4

Importance of Sexual
Pleasure in Life   5

Breaking the Taboo:
Discussing Sex
Positively   7

Chapter 2:
Communication in
Sexual Relationships   8

Importance of
Communication in
Sexual Relationships   8

How to Communicate
Your Sexual Desires   10

Active Listening:
Understanding Your
Partner's Sexual Desires   11

Chapter 3: The Art of
Foreplay   13

Why Foreplay is
Important   13

Different Types of
Foreplay   14

Tips and Techniques
for Better Foreplay   15

Chapter 4: Basic Sex
Positions   17

Missionary Position   17

Doggy Style   17

Cowgirl Position 17

Chapter 5: Intermediate
Sex Positions 17

Spooning Position 17

Reverse Cowgirl
Position 17

The Butterfly Position 17

Chapter 6: Advanced
Sex Positions 17

The Lotus Position 17

The G-Whiz Position 18

The Octopus Position 19

Chapter 7: Sex Toys and
Accessories 19

Introduction to Sex Toys 19

Different Types of Sex Toys 21

How to Use Sex Toys Safely 22

Chapter 8: Sexual Health and Safety 24

Importance of Sexual Health and Safety 24

Safe Sex Practices 25

Common Sexual Health Issues and Their Remedies 27

Chapter 9: Frequently Asked Questions 28

Answers to Common
Questions about Sex
Positions   28

Answers to Common
Questions about Sexual
Health and Safety   30

Chapter 10: Conclusion   31

Recap of Key Points   31

Final Thoughts and
Recommendations   33

Chapter 1: Introduction to Sexual Pleasure

Understanding Male Sexual Anatomy

Understanding Male Sexual Anatomy

To achieve maximum pleasure during sexual intercourse, it is important to understand the male sexual anatomy. The male sexual organ is known as the penis, which is made up of three main parts: the root, shaft, and glans.

The root is the base of the penis, where it attaches to the body. The shaft is the long, cylindrical part of the penis, while the glans is the rounded tip of the penis. The glans is also known as the head of the penis.

The penis is composed of spongy tissue that fills with blood during sexual arousal. This process, called an erection, allows the penis to become firm and engorged, making it ready for penetration during sexual intercourse.

The penis also has two main functions during sexual intercourse: ejaculation and urination. The urethra, which is a tube that runs through the penis, allows urine to exit the body. During ejaculation, semen is released through the urethra and out of the penis.

The male sexual anatomy also includes the testicles, which produce sperm and testosterone. The scrotum, which is a sac that hangs below the penis, holds the testicles and helps regulate their temperature.

It is important to note that every male's sexual anatomy varies in size, shape, and function. Some men may have a curved penis, while others may have a larger or smaller penis. It is important to embrace and understand your own unique anatomy and not compare yourself to others.

In order to have pleasurable and safe sexual experiences, it is important to practice good hygiene and use protection during sexual intercourse. This can include using condoms to prevent sexually transmitted infections and unwanted pregnancies.

Understanding male sexual anatomy is an important step in mastering sex positions and achieving maximum pleasure during sexual intercourse. By embracing and understanding your own unique anatomy, you can have pleasurable and safe sexual experiences.

Importance of Sexual Pleasure in Life

Sexual pleasure is an essential aspect of human life, and it has a significant impact on your overall well-being. As a young adult male, it is essential to understand the importance of sexual pleasure in life and how it can positively influence your life.

Firstly, sexual pleasure helps to reduce stress and anxiety. Engaging in sexual activities releases endorphins, which are natural mood enhancers. These endorphins help to lower stress levels and reduce anxiety, which can have a significant impact on your mental well-being. Additionally, sexual pleasure also helps to improve overall sleep quality, which is crucial for maintaining good health.

Secondly, sexual pleasure is a great way to improve your physical health. Engaging in sexual activities helps to increase blood flow, which can have a positive impact on your heart health. It also helps to improve your immune system, which can help to reduce the risk of getting sick.

Mastering Sex Positions: A Young Adult Male's Guide to Pleasure

Furthermore, sexual pleasure is an excellent way to build intimacy and strengthen relationships. Engaging in sexual activities with your partner helps to build trust, enhance communication, and create a deeper emotional connection. It is an excellent way to explore your partner's desires and create a stronger bond.

Lastly, sexual pleasure is a great way to explore your own sexuality and enhance self-confidence. Understanding your sexual preferences and desires can help you to become more confident in yourself and your sexuality. It can also help you to communicate your needs and desires to your partner, leading to a more fulfilling sexual experience.

Mastering Sex Positions: A Young Adult Male's Guide to Pleasure

To ensure maximum sexual pleasure, it is essential to explore different sex positions and techniques. The book "Mastering Sex Positions: A Young Adult Male's Guide to Pleasure" is an excellent resource for young adult males looking to enhance their sexual experience. It provides practical advice and guidance on various sex positions and techniques that can help to maximize pleasure and satisfaction.

In conclusion, sexual pleasure is an essential aspect of human life, and it has numerous benefits for your physical and mental well-being. As a young adult male, it is essential to explore your sexuality and understand the importance of sexual pleasure in life. The book "Mastering Sex Positions: A Young Adult Male's Guide to Pleasure" is an excellent resource to help you enhance your sexual experience and maximize pleasure.

Breaking the Taboo: Discussing Sex Positively

Breaking the Taboo: Discussing Sex Positively

Mastering Sex Positions: A Young Adult Male's Guide to Pleasure

Sex is a natural part of life that should be celebrated and enjoyed. Unfortunately, society often portrays sex as something taboo and shameful. This stigma can make it difficult for young adult males to talk openly about sex and explore their sexuality.

However, it's important to break this taboo and discuss sex positively. By doing so, we can create a healthier and more fulfilling sex life for ourselves and our partners. Here are some tips on how to discuss sex positively:

Mastering Sex Positions: A Young Adult Male's Guide to Pleasure

1. Be open and honest: Start by being open and honest with yourself about your sexual desires and preferences. Then, share these with your partner in a respectful and non-judgmental way. This can help strengthen your bond and lead to more satisfying sexual experiences.

2. Educate yourself: Educate yourself on sexual health and pleasure. Learn about different sex positions, techniques, and how to communicate with your partner. This knowledge can help you feel more confident and comfortable when discussing sex.

3. Listen actively: When discussing sex with your partner, make sure to listen actively and without judgment. This can help you understand their needs and desires, and lead to a more fulfilling sexual experience for both of you.

4. Communicate clearly: Communicate clearly and directly with your partner about what you want and what you're comfortable with. This can help avoid misunderstandings and ensure that both partners are on the same page.

5. Be respectful: Always respect your partner's boundaries and preferences. Don't pressure them into doing anything they're not comfortable with, and always ask for their consent before engaging in any sexual activity.

By breaking the taboo and discussing sex positively, we can create a more open and accepting society. This can lead to a healthier and more fulfilling sex life for everyone involved. So don't be afraid to talk openly about sex, and explore your sexuality in a safe and respectful manner.

Chapter 2: Communication in Sexual Relationships

Importance of Communication in Sexual Relationships

Sexual relationships are an essential part of any adult's life, and communication plays a crucial role in making it satisfying and pleasurable. The lack of communication leads to misunderstandings, discomfort, and dissatisfaction. It is vital to have open and honest communication with your partner about your sexual desires, needs, and preferences.

Communication in sexual relationships involves expressing your feelings, desires, and expectations to your partner. It is essential to be clear and concise about what you want and expect from the relationship, leaving no room for misunderstanding. Discussing sexual activities, positions, and fantasies can lead to a more satisfying experience for both partners.

Mastering Sex Positions: A Young Adult Male's Guide to Pleasure

Effective communication also involves listening to your partner's needs, desires, and preferences. It is crucial to be attentive and responsive to your partner's verbal and non-verbal cues. Understanding your partner's needs and desires will help you create a more intimate and pleasurable experience.

Moreover, communication in sexual relationships can improve the emotional connection between partners. It can lead to a deeper understanding of each other's emotions, which can enhance the bond between partners. Talking about your feelings and emotions during and after sexual activities can help you build trust and intimacy in your relationship.

Communication in sexual relationships is also essential for maintaining a healthy and safe sexual experience. It is crucial to discuss sexual health, including contraception, sexually transmitted infections (STIs), and HIV/AIDS. Having an open and honest conversation about these topics can help prevent the spread of STIs and ensure a healthy sexual experience.

In conclusion, communication is a vital aspect of sexual relationships. It is essential to have open and honest communication with your partner about your sexual desires, needs, and preferences. Effective communication can lead to a more satisfying sexual experience, improve the emotional connection between partners, and maintain a healthy and safe sexual experience.

How to Communicate Your Sexual Desires

As a young adult male, it's important to learn how to communicate your sexual desires in a healthy and respectful way. Whether it's with a new partner or someone you've been seeing for a while, expressing what you want in the bedroom can lead to more enjoyable and fulfilling sexual experiences for both parties.

Here are some tips on how to communicate your sexual desires effectively:

1. Be honest: It's important to be honest with your partner about what you want and what you don't want. This can be difficult if you're worried about hurting their feelings or being judged, but remember that communication is key to a healthy sexual relationship. Start the conversation by talking about what you enjoy about your current sexual experiences and then move on to discussing what you'd like to try.

2. Use "I" statements: When discussing your sexual desires, it's important to use "I" statements rather than "you" statements. This means focusing on your own feelings and desires rather than placing blame or making your partner feel like they're doing something wrong. For example, instead of saying "You never do this for me," try saying "I really enjoy when we do this together."

3. Be specific: When discussing your sexual desires, try to be as specific as possible. This can help your partner understand exactly what you want and can make it easier for them to fulfill your desires. For example, instead of saying "I want to try something new," try saying "I'd love to try this specific position or activity."

4. Listen to your partner: Communication is a two-way street, so it's important to listen to your partner's desires as well. Encourage them to share what they want and be open to trying new things together. Remember that sexual pleasure is a shared experience and it's important to prioritize your partner's needs and desires as well.

Overall, communicating your sexual desires can be intimidating, but it's an important part of building a healthy and fulfilling sexual relationship. Remember to be honest, use "I" statements, be specific, and listen to your partner to maximize pleasure for both parties.

Active Listening: Understanding Your Partner's Sexual Desires

Active Listening: Understanding Your Partner's Sexual Desires

Sexual desires are unique to every individual, and it is important that you understand your partner's sexual desires. Active listening is the key to understanding your partner's needs and wants in bed. When you actively listen to your partner, it shows that you care about their sexual satisfaction and pleasure. This chapter will guide you on how to actively listen to your partner and understand their sexual desires.

Pay Attention to Nonverbal Cues

Nonverbal cues can tell you a lot about your partner's sexual desires. You can observe your partner's breathing patterns, body movements, and facial expressions to know what they like or dislike during sex. If your partner moans, arches their back, or breathes heavily, these are signs that they are enjoying what you are doing. If they tense up or seem uncomfortable, it may be time to change positions or try something new.

Ask Questions

Asking questions is an excellent way to understand your partner's sexual desires. When you ask questions, you show that you are interested in what they want and that you want to make sure they are satisfied. You can ask questions like, "Do you like this position?" or "What can I do to make you feel more pleasure?" Be open to feedback and suggestions from your partner, and don't be afraid to communicate your own desires as well.

Try New Things

Trying new things in bed can be exciting and fun, but it is important to make sure that both you and your partner are comfortable with it. If you want to try something new, like a new sex position or a new sexual activity, talk to your partner about it first. Be respectful of their boundaries and listen to their concerns. If they are open to trying something new, start slow and communicate throughout the experience to make sure that both of you are enjoying it.

In conclusion, active listening is crucial to understanding your partner's sexual desires. Pay attention to nonverbal cues, ask questions, and try new things with respect and communication. By doing so, you can ensure that both you and your partner have a pleasurable and satisfying sexual experience.

Chapter 3: The Art of Foreplay

Why Foreplay is Important

Why Foreplay is Important

Foreplay is often considered as the warm-up before the main event. However, it is much more than that. Foreplay is an essential part of any sexual experience - it sets the tone for the entire encounter and can make or break the overall experience. As a young adult male, it's important to understand the importance of foreplay and how it can enhance your sexual pleasure.

Firstly, foreplay helps to build sexual tension and anticipation. It's the perfect opportunity to tease and explore each other's bodies before the main event. A good foreplay session can leave both partners craving more and can lead to a more intense and satisfying sexual experience.

Secondly, foreplay is crucial for women to reach orgasm. Unlike men, women's bodies take longer to become fully aroused, and foreplay is the perfect way to get her in the mood. Foreplay allows time for the clitoris to become engorged and for the vaginal walls to lubricate, making penetration more comfortable and pleasurable.

Thirdly, foreplay is a great way to explore each other's bodies and discover what turns your partner on. This can be a fun and exciting experience, allowing you to try out new techniques and positions that you may not have considered before.

Finally, foreplay is an excellent opportunity to build intimacy and emotional connection with your partner. It's a chance to slow down and focus on each other, creating a deeper level of trust and understanding.

In conclusion, foreplay is an essential part of any sexual experience. It sets the tone for the encounter, helps women reach orgasm, allows for exploration and discovery, and builds intimacy and emotional connection. As a young adult male, taking the time to engage in foreplay will not only enhance your sexual pleasure but also lead to a more satisfying and fulfilling sexual experience for both you and your partner.

Different Types of Foreplay

Foreplay is an essential aspect of sex that is often overlooked by young adult males. While sex positions garner a lot of attention, foreplay sets the stage for an enjoyable and satisfying sexual experience. In this subchapter, we will explore the different types of foreplay that can help you and your partner achieve maximum pleasure.

Mastering Sex Positions: A Young Adult Male's Guide to Pleasure

1. Kissing: Kissing is a classic form of foreplay that never goes out of style. Whether it's a gentle peck on the lips or a passionate make-out session, kissing can ignite the flames of desire and get you in the mood for more.

2. Touching: Touching is another essential form of foreplay that involves exploring your partner's body with your hands. Gently caressing their skin, running your fingers through their hair, and touching their erogenous zones can all contribute to a heightened sense of arousal.

3. Oral sex: Oral sex is a popular form of foreplay that involves stimulating your partner's genitals with your mouth. Whether it's giving or receiving, oral sex can be a highly enjoyable and intimate experience that can bring you and your partner closer together.

4. Massage: A sensual massage can be a great way to relax and unwind before sex. Using a massage oil or lotion, you can gently rub your partner's body, paying special attention to their erogenous zones, to help them relax and prepare for more intimate activities.

5. Dirty talk: Sometimes, words can be just as arousing as physical touch. Dirty talk involves using sexually explicit language to describe your desires and fantasies, which can help you and your partner get in the mood for more intimate activities.

In summary, foreplay is an essential aspect of sex that can help you and your partner achieve maximum pleasure. By exploring different types of foreplay, such as kissing, touching, oral sex, massage, and dirty talk, you can heighten your sexual experience and create a deeper connection with your partner. Remember, sex is not just about the destination but the journey, so take your time and enjoy the ride.

Tips and Techniques for Better Foreplay

Foreplay is an essential part of any sexual encounter and can greatly enhance the pleasure experienced during sex. Many young adult males often overlook the importance of foreplay and jump straight into penetration, but taking the time to engage in foreplay can lead to a more satisfying and enjoyable sexual experience for both partners.

Here are some tips and techniques for better foreplay:

1. Start Slowly: Foreplay is not something that should be rushed. Take your time to explore your partner's body and find out what they enjoy. Kiss, touch, and caress them slowly, building up the sexual tension.

2. Communicate: Effective communication is essential in any sexual encounter. Ask your partner what they like and what they don't like. This will help you to tailor your foreplay to their specific desires.

3. Use Your Hands: Your hands are a powerful tool when it comes to foreplay. Use them to touch and caress your partner's erogenous zones, such as their neck, ears, nipples, and inner thighs.

4. Incorporate Oral Sex: Oral sex can be a highly enjoyable form of foreplay for both partners. Experiment with different techniques, such as licking, sucking, and nibbling, to find out what your partner enjoys.

5. Try Different Positions: Foreplay doesn't have to be limited to just one position. Experiment with different positions, such as standing, sitting, or lying down, to keep things interesting.

6. Use Toys: Sex toys can be a great addition to foreplay. Incorporating a vibrator or dildo can help to enhance your partner's pleasure and lead to a more intense orgasm.

7. Don't Forget About Kissing: Kissing is a highly intimate and erotic act that should not be overlooked during foreplay. Take the time to kiss your partner passionately and explore their mouth with your tongue.

In conclusion, foreplay is an essential part of any sexual encounter and should not be overlooked. By taking the time to engage in foreplay and experimenting with different techniques and positions, you can greatly enhance the pleasure experienced during sex and lead to a more satisfying sexual encounter for both partners.

Chapter 4: Basic Sex Positions

Missionary Position

Doggy Style

Cowgirl Position

Chapter 5: Intermediate Sex Positions

Spooning Position

Reverse Cowgirl Position

The Butterfly Position

Chapter 6: Advanced Sex Positions

The Lotus Position

The G-Whiz Position

The G-Whiz Position

The G-Whiz position is a popular sex position that is designed to stimulate the G-spot in women. This position is highly recommended for couples who want to enhance their sexual experience and achieve intense orgasms.

Mastering Sex Positions: A Young Adult Male's Guide to Pleasure

To perform the G-Whiz position, the male partner must lie on his back and bend his knees while keeping his feet flat on the bed. The female partner must straddle him, facing him, with her knees bent and feet flat on the bed. She must then lean back and use her hands to support her weight while arching her back. The male partner can use his hands to support her hips and guide her movements.

One of the key benefits of the G-Whiz position is that it allows for deeper penetration, which can stimulate the G-spot and provide intense orgasms for women. Additionally, this position allows for easy access to the clitoris, which can be stimulated manually or with a vibrator.

Mastering Sex Positions: A Young Adult Male's Guide to Pleasure

Couples who want to try the G-Whiz position should take their time and communicate with each other throughout the process. It is important to find a comfortable angle and depth of penetration that works for both partners. Additionally, couples should experiment with different speeds and movements to find what feels pleasurable.

It is also important to note that not all women may experience intense orgasms from G-spot stimulation. Some women may need additional clitoral stimulation to achieve orgasm. Therefore, couples should be open to exploring different combinations of stimulation to find what works best for them.

In conclusion, the G-Whiz position is a popular sex position that can enhance sexual pleasure for couples. While it is not a guarantee for intense orgasms, it is worth trying for couples who want to experiment and explore new ways to enjoy their sexual experiences. Remember to communicate with your partner, take your time, and have fun!

The Octopus Position

Chapter 7: Sex Toys and Accessories

Introduction to Sex Toys

Introduction to Sex Toys

Mastering Sex Positions: A Young Adult Male's Guide to Pleasure

Sex toys are becoming increasingly popular among young adults. They are a great way to enhance sexual pleasure and explore new sensations. In this chapter, we will introduce you to some of the most popular sex toys and provide you with tips on how to use them.

But first, let's answer the question, what is a sex toy? A sex toy is an object or device designed to enhance sexual pleasure. They come in a variety of shapes, sizes, and materials, and can be used alone or with a partner.

Now, let's get into the different types of sex toys.

1. Vibrators – Vibrators are the most popular sex toy for women. They come in a variety of shapes and sizes and can be used for both clitoral and vaginal stimulation. Some vibrators even have different vibration patterns and intensities to explore.

2. Dildos – Dildos are penis-shaped sex toys that can be used for vaginal or anal penetration. They come in a variety of sizes and materials, including silicone, glass, and metal.

3. Butt plugs – Butt plugs are sex toys designed for anal play. They come in a variety of sizes and shapes, and can be used alone or with a partner.

4. Cock rings – Cock rings are sex toys that are worn around the base of the penis. They help to maintain an erection and enhance sexual pleasure.

5. Fleshlights – Fleshlights are male masturbators that are designed to look and feel like a vagina. They come in a variety of textures and can be used for solo play or with a partner.

When using sex toys, it's important to remember to always use lube. This will help to prevent any discomfort or pain. Also, make sure to clean your sex toys after each use to prevent the spread of bacteria.

In conclusion, sex toys are a great way to enhance sexual pleasure and explore new sensations. With so many different types of sex toys available, there is something for everyone. Just remember to always use lube, clean your sex toys, and most importantly, have fun!

Different Types of Sex Toys

Different Types of Sex Toys

Sex toys have been around for centuries and have evolved over time. They come in different shapes, sizes, and materials. In this chapter, we will discuss the different types of sex toys that you can explore to enhance your sexual experiences.

1. Vibrators

Vibrators are the most popular sex toys for women. They are designed to stimulate the clitoris, vagina, or both. Vibrators come in different shapes and sizes, from bullet vibes to rabbit vibes. Bullet vibes are small and discreet, while rabbit vibes are larger and have a rabbit-shaped extension that stimulates the clitoris.

2. Dildos

Dildos are designed to mimic the shape and size of the penis. They come in different materials, including silicone, glass, and metal. Some dildos have a suction cup at the base for hands-free play, while others have a harness attachment for strap-on play.

3. Anal Toys

Anal toys are designed to stimulate the anus. They come in different shapes and sizes, from butt plugs to anal beads. Butt plugs are designed to stay in place, while anal beads are designed for insertion and removal.

4. Cock Rings

Cock rings are designed to enhance erections and prolong ejaculation. They come in different materials, including silicone and metal. Some cock rings have a vibrating attachment for added stimulation.

5. BDSM Toys

BDSM toys are designed for bondage and domination play. They come in different materials, including leather and metal. Some BDSM toys include handcuffs, whips, and restraints.

6. Fleshlights

Fleshlights are designed to mimic the sensation of vaginal or anal sex. They come in different shapes and sizes, and some are designed to look like a real vagina or anus.

In conclusion, sex toys can enhance your sexual experiences and add a new level of excitement to your sex life. It's important to choose a sex toy that suits your preferences and comfort level. Experimenting with different types of sex toys can help you discover new ways to pleasure yourself and your partner.

How to Use Sex Toys Safely

Sex toys are becoming increasingly popular among couples and singles alike, providing an exciting way to add some variety and spice to your sex life. However, with this added excitement comes the need for responsibility and safety. Here are some tips for using sex toys safely and effectively:

1. Choose Quality Products

When selecting sex toys, it's essential to choose products made from high-quality materials. Low-quality sex toys can contain dangerous chemicals and toxins that can be harmful to your health. Always read the label and research the manufacturer before making a purchase.

2. Clean Your Toys Regularly

Proper hygiene is essential when it comes to sex toys. Always clean your toys before and after use to prevent the spread of bacteria and infection. Use a mild soap and warm water to clean your toys, and make sure to dry them thoroughly before storing them.

3. Use Lubrication

Using lubrication can make sex toy play more comfortable and enjoyable. However, it's important to choose the right type of lubricant for your toy. For example, silicone-based lubricants can damage silicone toys, so it's best to use water-based lubricants instead.

4. Be Careful with Anal Toys

Anal toys can be a great way to explore new sensations, but it's essential to use them safely. Always use a water-based lubricant, and start with smaller toys before moving on to larger ones. Never share anal toys with multiple partners, as this can increase the risk of infection.

5. Store Your Toys Properly

Proper storage is crucial when it comes to sex toys. Keep them in a clean, dry place, and store them separately from other toys to prevent contamination. Avoid leaving them in direct sunlight or extreme heat, as this can damage the material.

In conclusion, using sex toys can be a fun and exciting way to explore your sexuality, but it's essential to do so safely. By following these tips and using common sense, you can enjoy your toys without putting your health at risk.

Chapter 8: Sexual Health and Safety

Importance of Sexual Health and Safety

Mastering Sex Positions: A Young Adult Male's Guide to Pleasure

Sexual health and safety are two essential aspects that young adult males need to understand to ensure they enjoy a fulfilling sex life. It is crucial to understand that sexual health goes beyond just preventing sexually transmitted infections (STIs) and unwanted pregnancies. It involves taking care of your physical, emotional, and mental well-being when engaging in sexual activities. By prioritizing sexual health and safety, you can enjoy a pleasurable and safe sex life.

The following are the reasons why sexual health and safety are important:

1. Protection against STIs and unwanted pregnancies

Using condoms and other forms of protection during sexual activities reduces the risk of contracting STIs and unwanted pregnancies. It is crucial to use protection consistently and correctly to ensure maximum protection.

2. Prevention of sexual assault

Consent is vital in any sexual encounter. Young adult males need to understand the importance of obtaining consent before engaging in any sexual activity. It is also essential to respect your partner's boundaries and communicate effectively to avoid any misunderstandings.

3. Emotional well-being

Sexual activities can significantly impact one's emotional well-being. It is essential to engage in sexual activities with someone you trust and respect to avoid feeling emotionally drained or used.

4. Mental health

Sexual activities can significantly affect one's mental health. It is important to understand the potential risks associated with sex, such as addiction, depression, and anxiety. Young adult males need to prioritize their mental health and seek help if they experience any negative effects associated with sex.

In conclusion, sexual health and safety are vital aspects that young adult males need to prioritize when engaging in sexual activities. By understanding the importance of protection, consent, emotional well-being, and mental health, you can enjoy a pleasurable and safe sex life. It is crucial to educate yourself on sexual health and safety to avoid any potential risks and have a fulfilling sexual experience.

Safe Sex Practices

Safe Sex Practices

Mastering Sex Positions: A Young Adult Male's Guide to Pleasure

When it comes to sex, it's important to prioritize your health and safety. Not only can unsafe sex lead to unwanted pregnancies, but it can also put you at risk for sexually transmitted infections (STIs). Here are some safe sex practices to keep in mind:

1. Use protection: Always use a condom when engaging in sexual activity, especially if you are not in a monogamous relationship. Condoms can help prevent the transmission of STIs and protect against unwanted pregnancies.

2. Get tested: It's important to get tested for STIs regularly, even if you don't have any symptoms. This can help you identify and treat any potential infections early on.

3. Talk to your partner: Communication is key when it comes to safe sex. Talk to your partner about their sexual history and any potential risks before engaging in sexual activity.

4. Avoid alcohol and drugs: Substance abuse can impair your judgment and increase your likelihood of engaging in risky sexual behavior. It's important to stay sober and make informed decisions about your sexual health.

5. Practice good hygiene: Keeping yourself clean and maintaining good hygiene can help prevent the transmission of STIs. Be sure to shower regularly and wash your hands before and after sexual activity.

Remember, safe sex is important for both your physical and emotional well-being. By practicing safe sex, you can enjoy a fulfilling sex life while also protecting yourself and your partner from potential risks.

Common Sexual Health Issues and Their Remedies

Sexual health is an important aspect of overall well-being and pleasure. As a young adult male, you may encounter various sexual health issues that may affect your ability to enjoy sex, such as erectile dysfunction, premature ejaculation, and low libido. Fortunately, there are remedies for these common sexual health issues that can help you improve your sexual performance and pleasure.

Erectile dysfunction (ED) is a common sexual health issue that affects many men. It occurs when you have trouble getting or maintaining an erection during sexual activity. ED can be caused by various factors, such as stress, anxiety, depression, or physical health problems such as diabetes, high blood pressure, or heart disease. To remedy ED, you can try various treatments such as medication, counseling, lifestyle changes, or natural remedies like herbal supplements.

Premature ejaculation (PE) is another common sexual health issue that can affect your sexual performance. It occurs when you ejaculate too quickly during sexual activity, before you or your partner is ready. PE can be caused by psychological factors such as anxiety, stress, or relationship issues, or physical factors such as hormonal imbalances or nerve damage. To remedy PE, you can try various techniques such as the squeeze method, the stop-start method, or medication.

Low libido is a sexual health issue that can affect your desire for sex. It occurs when you have a decreased interest in sexual activity, and it can be caused by various factors such as stress, fatigue, depression, or hormonal imbalances. To remedy low libido, you can try various techniques such as lifestyle changes, counseling, or medication.

In conclusion, sexual health issues can be a barrier to enjoying sex to the fullest. However, by understanding the causes and remedies for common sexual health issues, you can improve your sexual performance and pleasure. Whether you are dealing with ED, PE, or low libido, there are various treatments and techniques that can help you overcome these issues and enjoy a fulfilling sex life.

Chapter 9: Frequently Asked Questions

Answers to Common Questions about Sex Positions

Answers to Common Questions about Sex

Positions

When it comes to sex, one of the most exciting

things about it is the variety of positions you can

try out. However, with so many options available,

it's common to have questions about the best

way to approach certain positions. Here are some

answers to some of the most common questions

about sex positions.

Q: What are some good positions for beginners?

A: If you're new to sex, it's best to start with positions that are simple and easy to master. Missionary is a classic position that allows you to make eye contact and easily control the pace and depth of penetration. Doggy style is another popular option that allows for deeper penetration and allows both partners to enjoy a more animalistic experience.

Q: What are some positions for deeper penetration?

A: If you're looking to go deeper, try positions like missionary with legs raised or modified doggy style where the receiving partner is on their stomach with their hips raised. Also, the cowgirl position can be a great option for deeper penetration as the receiving partner can control the angle and depth of penetration.

Q: Are there positions that are better for clitoral stimulation?

A: Yes! Positions like woman on top and reverse cowgirl allow for greater clitoral stimulation as the receiving partner has more control over the angle and pressure of stimulation.

Q: Can sex positions help with premature ejaculation?

A: Yes, certain positions can help with premature ejaculation. Positions like the stop and start method, where the thrusting is stopped periodically, can help you last longer. Additionally, positions that allow for slower, more controlled movements like spooning or missionary with legs wrapped around can allow you to last longer.

Q: What are some positions for anal sex?

A: Anal sex requires more preparation and care, but there are several positions that can make it more comfortable and enjoyable. Doggy style and reverse cowgirl are popular positions for anal sex, as they allow for deeper penetration and more control over the angle of penetration.

Remember, the most important thing when it comes to sex positions is finding what works best for you and your partner. Don't be afraid to experiment and try new things. With practice and communication, you can master any position and enjoy a fulfilling sex life.

Answers to Common Questions about Sexual Health and Safety

Answers to Common Questions about Sexual Health and Safety

Sexual health and safety are crucial aspects of any sexual encounter. However, many young adult males often have questions and concerns about these topics. Here are some answers to common questions about sexual health and safety.

Q: How do I know if I have an STD?

A: The only way to know for sure if you have an STD is to get tested. Symptoms of STDs can vary, and some people may not have any symptoms at all. It's important to get tested regularly, especially if you are sexually active with multiple partners.

Q: What are some ways to prevent STDs?

A: The most effective way to prevent STDs is to use condoms consistently and correctly during sexual activity. It's also important to limit sexual partners and get tested regularly.

Q: Is it safe to have sex during a woman's period?

A: It is safe to have sex during a woman's period, but there may be an increased risk of infection. It's important to use protection and practice good hygiene to reduce the risk of infection.

Mastering Sex Positions: A Young Adult Male's Guide to Pleasure

Q: Can I get pregnant if I have sex during my partner's period?

A: It is possible to get pregnant if you have sex during your partner's period. Sperm can survive for up to five days in the female reproductive system, so it's important to use protection if you don't want to get pregnant.

Q: How do I know if I'm ready to have sex?

A: It's important to make sure that you are emotionally and mentally ready to have sex. You should also make sure that you are prepared to practice safe sex and communicate with your partner about your boundaries and expectations.

In summary, sexual health and safety are essential aspects of any sexual encounter. It's important to understand the risks and take steps to prevent STDs and unwanted pregnancies. Remember to communicate with your partner and practice safe sex to ensure a pleasurable and safe sexual experience.

Chapter 10: Conclusion

Recap of Key Points

Recap of Key Points:

Throughout this book, we've covered a variety of sex positions and techniques to enhance your pleasure and that of your partner. Here is a recap of some of the key points that we've discussed:

Mastering Sex Positions: A Young Adult Male's Guide to Pleasure

1. Communication is key: Whether you're trying a new position or exploring new fantasies, it's important to communicate with your partner. Discuss your likes, dislikes, and boundaries to avoid any misunderstandings.

2. Foreplay is essential: Foreplay is a crucial part of any sexual experience. Take the time to explore your partner's body, try different techniques, and build anticipation before moving on to intercourse.

3. Experiment with different positions: There are countless sex positions to try, and it's important to find what works best for you and your partner. Don't be afraid to try new things and mix things up to keep things exciting.

4. Pay attention to your partner's pleasure: Sex is not just about your pleasure, but also about your partner's. Pay attention to their reactions and adjust accordingly to ensure that they're enjoying themselves as well.

5. Use lube: Lube can enhance the pleasure and reduce discomfort during sex. Don't be afraid to use it, even if you don't think you need it.

6. Practice safe sex: Always use condoms and practice safe sex to protect yourself and your partner from sexually transmitted infections.

7. Don't be afraid to ask for help: If you're experiencing any sexual issues or have questions about sex, don't hesitate to ask for help. There are many resources available, including sex therapists, doctors, and online communities.

Remember, sex should be a pleasurable and enjoyable experience for both you and your partner. By being open to new experiences, communicating effectively, and being attentive to your partner's pleasure, you can master sex positions and enhance your sexual experiences.

Final Thoughts and Recommendations

As we come to the end of this book, I hope you have found it to be a helpful guide in exploring different sex positions and enhancing your sexual pleasure. In this final subchapter, I would like to share some final thoughts and recommendations that I believe will help you take your sexual experiences to the next level.

Firstly, I want to emphasize the importance of communication in any sexual relationship. It is crucial to talk openly and honestly with your partner about what feels good and what doesn't, what you want to try and what you're not comfortable with. This will not only help you both enjoy the experience more but will also strengthen your relationship outside of the bedroom.

Secondly, I want to remind you that sex is not just about penetration or reaching orgasm. It's about exploring each other's bodies, finding what turns each other on and enjoying the experience together. So don't be fixated on trying to achieve a certain position or goal, but rather focus on connecting with your partner and exploring each other's desires.

Lastly, I want to recommend that you continue to educate yourself on sex and sexuality. There is always something new to learn or try, and the more you know, the more you can experiment and enjoy. There are many resources available, from books and articles to online communities and workshops. Don't be afraid to seek out information and explore new ideas.

Mastering Sex Positions: A Young Adult Male's Guide to Pleasure

In conclusion, I hope this book has been a helpful guide in mastering different sex positions and exploring your sexual pleasure. Remember to communicate with your partner, focus on the experience and continue to educate yourself. With these tools, you can create a fulfilling and satisfying sexual relationship that will bring pleasure and joy for years to come.

Mastering Sex Positions: A Young Adult Male's Guide to Pleasure

Thanks for reading! Best of luck, skill, and love in your sex life - Kelly :)